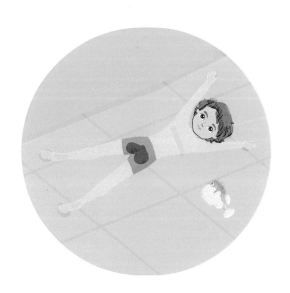

Learn to Swim the Australian Way
Level 1 Foundations
Written by AlyT

Learn To Swim the Australian Way
Level 1 Foundations

Part of the Learn to Swim The Australian Way series with AlyT

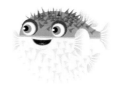

DEDICATED TO

my mother **RHONDA** aka **MRS PAUL**
who taught me everything I needed to know
about life & Jesus †

AND my mentor **PETER TIBBS** aka **TIBBSIE**; both
of whom helped mould me into the swimmer and
swimming teacher I am today.

Formatting: Aluycia Suceng
Editing: Jessie Raymond
Illustrator: PicassoJR
First printing: 2021

Disclaimer
While we draw on our own prior professional expertise and background in the area
of teaching learn to swim, by purchasing and reading our products you acknowledge
that we have produced this book for informational and educational purposes only. You
alone are solely responsible, and take full responsibility for your own wellbeing as well
as the health, lives and wellbeing of your family and children in your care.

www.BornToSwim.com.au
SwimMechanics@yahoo.com
Other books in our Welcome to Water Awareness Series include:
Water Awareness Newborn Infants
Water Awareness Babies
Water Awareness Toddlers

SAFETY FIRST!

* NEVER SWIM ALONE

The non-swimmer should always be accompanied by a responsible adult who can swim. Where possible, let the lifeguard on duty know you are learning to swim or a beginner swimmer.

* NEVER FORCE A SWIMMER UNDER THE WATER

Learning to swim should be fun & appropriate to the individual's pace. Whilst not ideal, many activities can be practised with the face out of the water until the nervous swimmer is ready to put their face under the water.

* NEVER HOLD YOUR BREATH FOR EXTENDED PERIODS OF TIME

Hyperventilating and breath holding games are dangerous and can cause you to faint (lose consciousness) in the water. Search 'shallow water black-out' for more information.

* LEARNING TO SWIM IN SHALLOW, WAIST DEPTH WATER IS BEST FOR BEGINNERS

Until you can confidently move yourself through the water and float comfortably on your back, beginner swimmers should continue to practise in shallow water only.

A NOTE TO ALL THE BUOYS & GULLS LEARNING TO SWIM,

Welcome to **LEARN TO SWIM THE AUSTRALIAN WAY: THE FOUNDATIONS**

Learning to swim is an accumulation of skills which need to be repeatedly practiced to perfection to **BUILD MUSCLE MEMORY, IMPROVE BALANCE** and **INCREASE THE TRACTION & PROPULSION** of the swimmer in the water. In this book we've used the building block method of skill progressions to work towards achieving these three goals.

This means each of the four strokes **(FREESTYLE, BACKSTROKE, BREASTSTROKE AND BUTTERFLY)**, dives, tumble turns, water safety etc have been broken down into their simplest form to ensure swimmers learn **EVERY PIECE OF THE TECHNICAL PUZZLE** that is swimming.

We also encourage the three P's of learning. **PATIENCE, PERFECTION & PRACTICE.** Some skills can be learnt in minutes, others may take weeks and months. All learner swimmers should follow the motto **LEARN SLOW TO SWIM FAST.**

Failing to learn a skill, moving too quickly through the learning of a skill and the continual practice of a poorly executed skill, with no regard to correcting mistakes, leads to bad habits and sloppy swimming. Level 1 learners should practice new skills over **SHORT DISTANCES OF 2-3 METERS IN SHALLOW WATER**; practicing newly learnt skills over longer distances leads to fatigue and the swimmers' new skills and technique will tend to fall apart.

Where possible, ensure the swimmer performs each skill to the best of their ability **4-5 TIMES EVERY LESSON**, don't be afraid to correct mistakes and remember to give **LOTS OF PRAISE AND ENCOURAGEMENT**. Each time a specific skill is practised the aim is to move toward perfect mastery of that particular skill. Keep in mind, the words 'I can't' do not exist in the learner swimmer's vocabulary, but **I'LL TRY AND A BIT OF EFFORT** always should.

For easy learning, this book includes **VISUAL CUES, CATCHY NAMES** and easy to remember **VERBAL CUES** for each skill, which we have presented **IN THE LOGICAL ORDER** as we would perform them during a real-time in-person class.

Our hope is parents and teachers will slowly progress through each skill, as either a guide to learning to swim at home or to compliment the structured lessons learnt at a professional swim school.

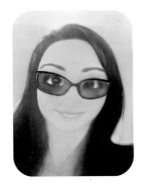

Yours swimmingly,

Alyt

P.S The quickest way to improve your swimming is to spend more time in the water, therefore we suggest practising at least 3x a week. Once each of the skills have been perfected, move on to the next learn to swim level in our series.

I CAN SAFELY ENTER THE WATER!

I never enter the water **without an adult** who can swim.

Once I know it is safe, I sit on the edge of the pool deck with my feet in the water. I place both hands beside me, then turn my body and slowly lower myself into the pool, making sure I hold on securely to the side of the pool.

Before entering the water I first check:

1 the depth of the water?

2 is there a safe place for me to get in and out of the water?

3 is someone watching and close by to help me if I need them?

I always walk, never run, as I approach the water slowly and carefully.

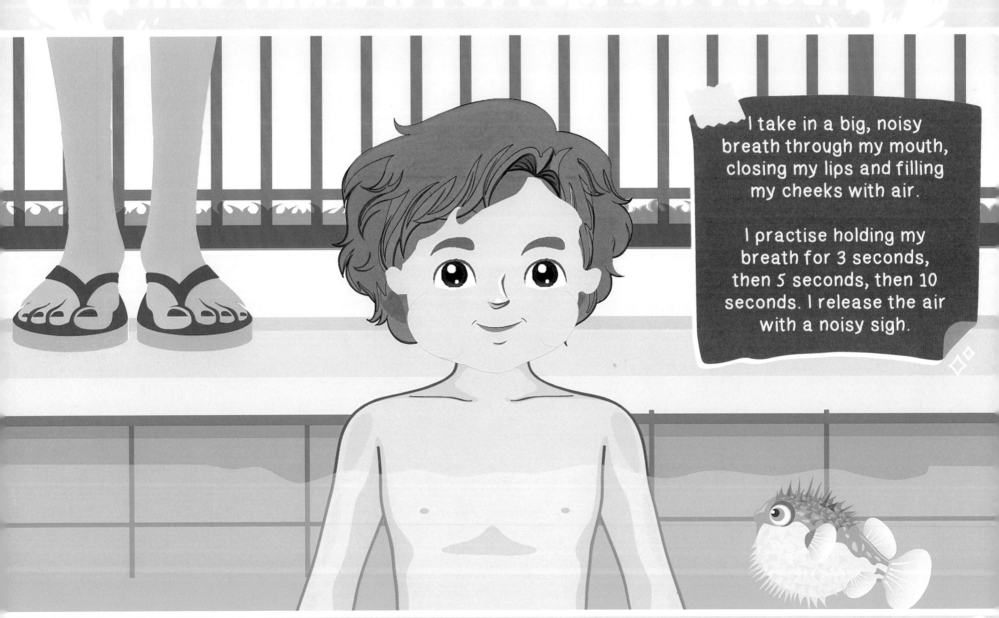

I CAN HOLD MY BREATH AND MAKE A PUFFERFISH FACE!

I take in a big, noisy breath through my mouth, closing my lips and filling my cheeks with air.

I practise holding my breath for 3 seconds, then 5 seconds, then 10 seconds. I release the air with a noisy sigh.

I CAN SUBMERGE MY WHOLE FACE UNDER THE WATER!

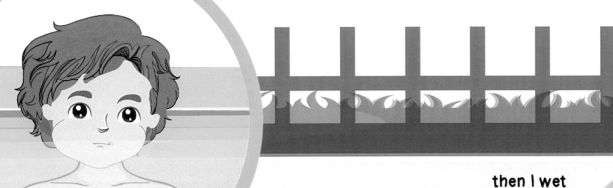

If I am nervous, I start by just wetting my shoulders and my chin,

then I wet both my ears one at a time.

I practise putting my face in for 5 seconds then lift my face out of the water. After a few tries, I can hold my breath and submerge my face for 1.2.3.4.5.6.7.8.9.10!

When I am ready, I take in a big, pufferfish breath and press my face into the water. I hold it there and look at my toes as I count to 3.

I CAN **BOB UP AND DOWN** TO GRAB A BREATH OF FRESH AIR!

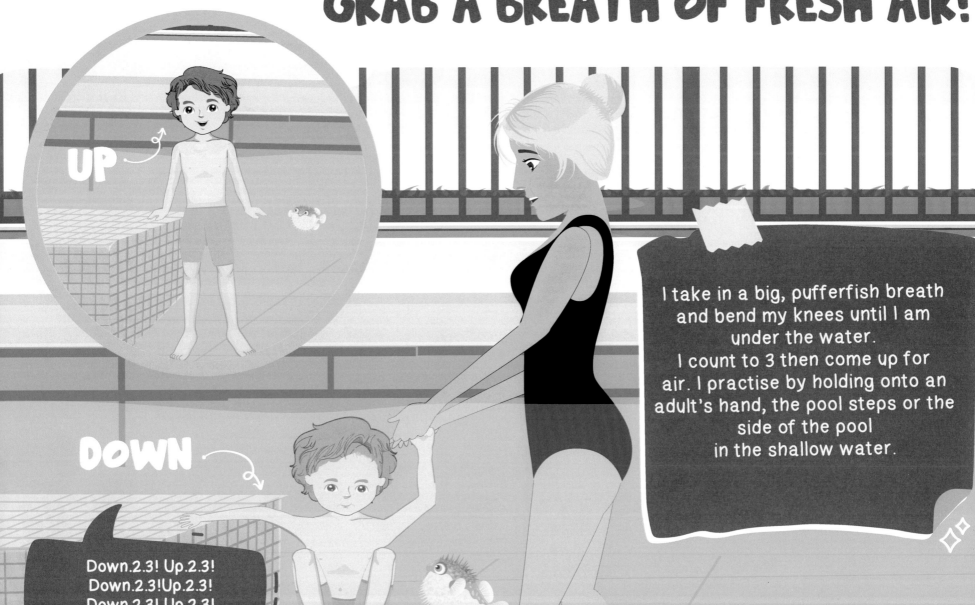

UP

DOWN

I take in a big, pufferfish breath and bend my knees until I am under the water.
I count to 3 then come up for air. I practise by holding onto an adult's hand, the pool steps or the side of the pool in the shallow water.

Down.2.3! Up.2.3!
Down.2.3!Up.2.3!
Down.2.3! Up.2.3!
HAVE A REST.

I CAN CROCODILE WALK ACROSS THE POOL FLOOR!

I stretch out long and flat in the shallow water and let my legs float up behind me. I point my toes and keep my ankles dry as I lift and lower my face into the water for a breath of fresh air, pulling myself through the water, using only my outstretched arms.

CROCODILE WALK

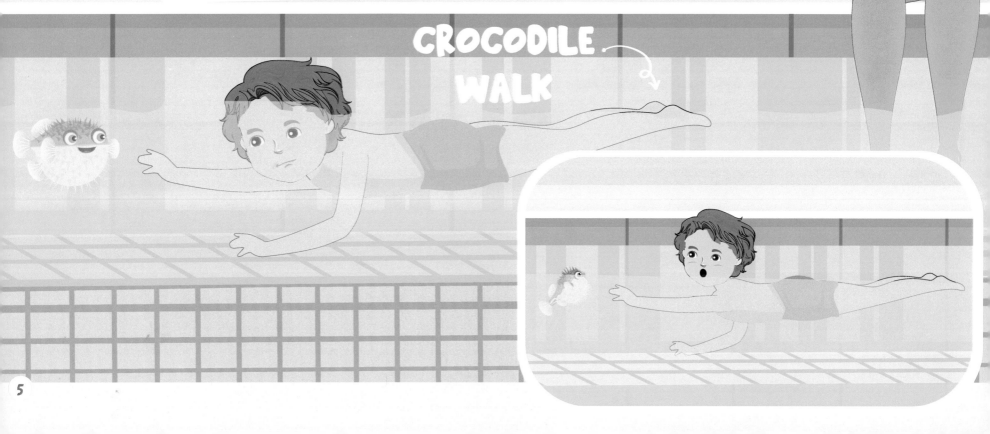

I CAN CROCODILE HOLD THE KICKBOARD!

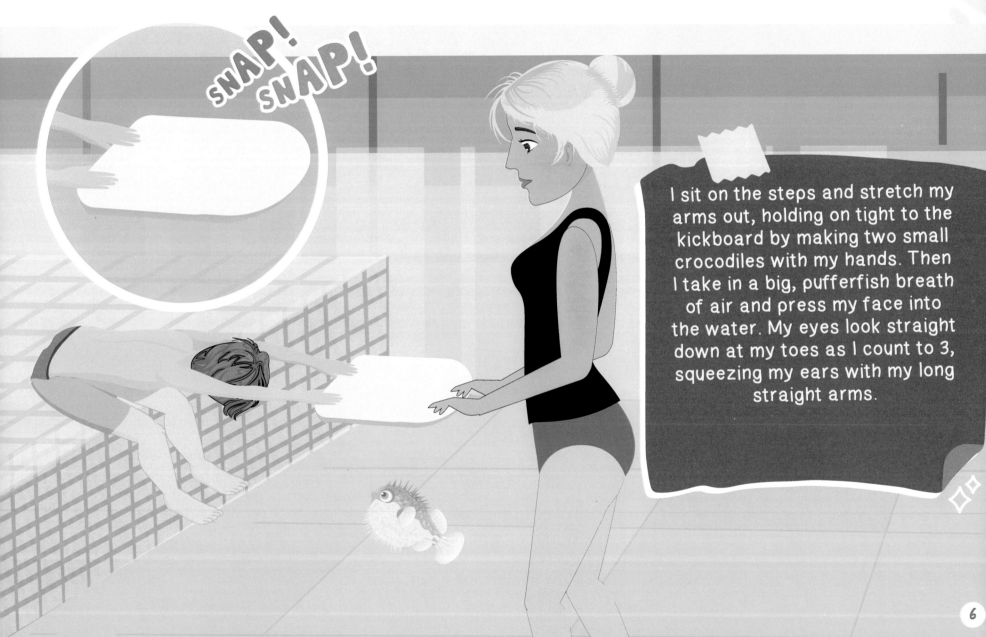

SNAP! SNAP!

I sit on the steps and stretch my arms out, holding on tight to the kickboard by making two small crocodiles with my hands. Then I take in a big, pufferfish breath of air and press my face into the water. My eyes look straight down at my toes as I count to 3, squeezing my ears with my long straight arms.

I CAN STARFISH FLOAT ON MY BELLY!

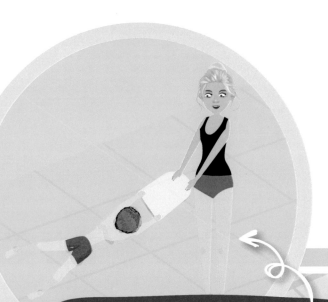

To stand back up, I lift my head and bend my knees to my chest so I can plant my feet back on the pool floor.

I learn my starfish floats by first holding onto a kickboard with the help of an adult. I take in a big, pufferfish breath and press my face into the water. I look straight down and let my legs float behind me, pointing my toes and keeping my ankles dry. When I am ready, I do a starfish float without the kickboard.

Lift Head

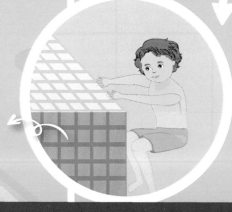

Plant feet

I start by sitting or standing in the pool and spreading my arms into the shape of a Y. I keep my arms straight and wide, as I hold my pufferfish breath and look at the bottom of the pool. My legs stretch out behind me and I point my toes. I lay flat on the water in the shape of a star and feel the water gently holding me. I relax as I count to 10.

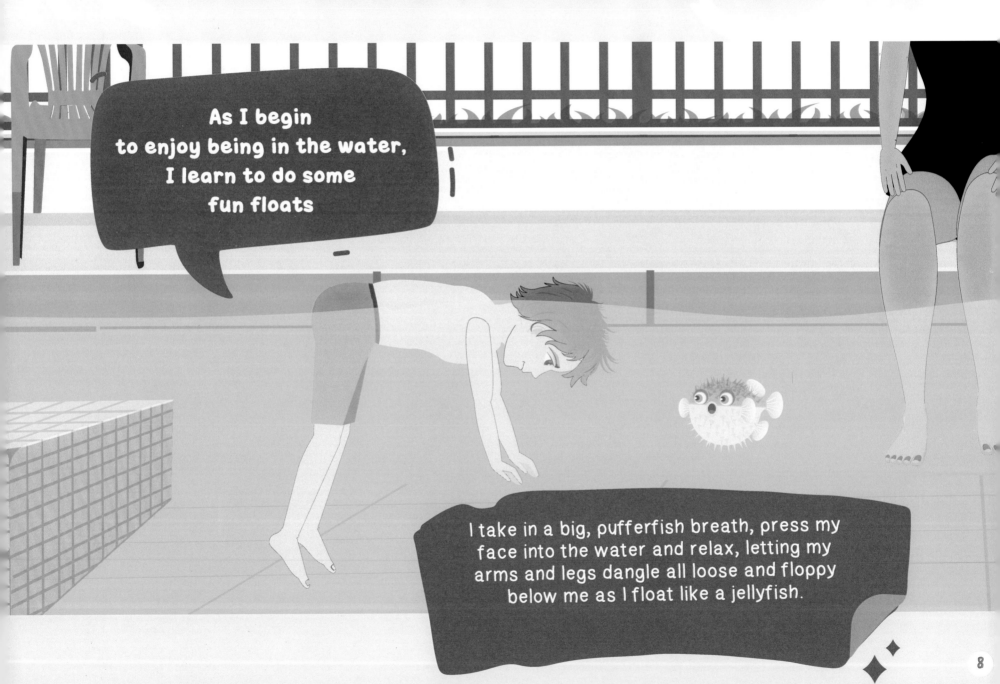

I CAN MARSHMALLOW FLOAT!

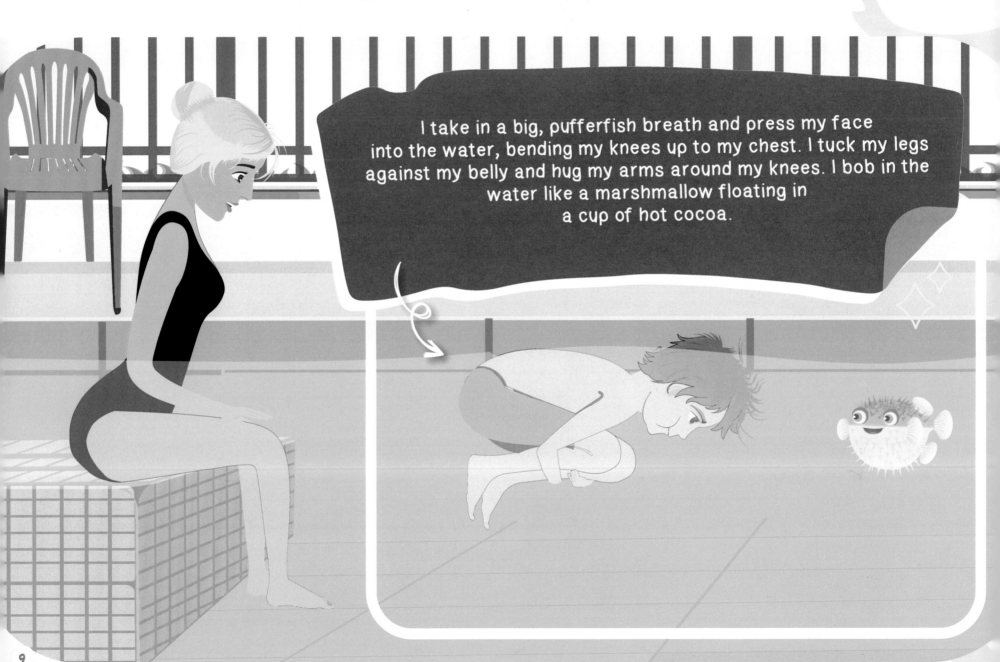

I take in a big, pufferfish breath and press my face into the water, bending my knees up to my chest. I tuck my legs against my belly and hug my arms around my knees. I bob in the water like a marshmallow floating in a cup of hot cocoa.

I CAN TEDDY BEAR HUG THE KICKBOARD

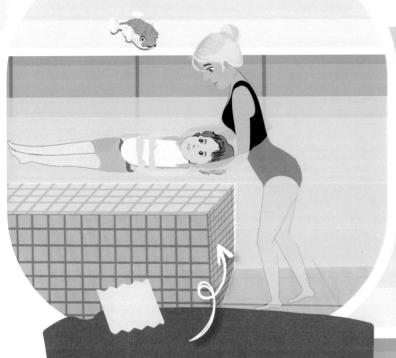

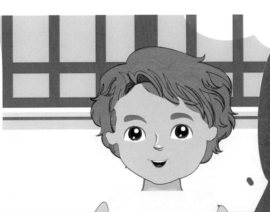

I start by putting the kickboard on my chest under my chin and wrap my arms around it like I am giving it a soft hug.

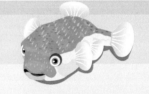

To practice my backfloat, I sit in the shallow water and slowly lay myself down flat, with my ears under the water, as I hug the kickboard. I look straight up at the sky and relax as the water gently laps around me. The water sometimes tickles my ears, but it comes out when I finish my float.

I learn to cuddle the kickboard so I can back float. The kickboard will help me stay afloat while I learn to relax and lay on my back in the water. An adult will help me until I can do it by myself.

I CAN STARFISH FLOAT ON MY BACK!

Head back ears under

To stand back up, I lift my head and look at my feet. Then I bend my knees to my chest, sitting up in the water and planting my feet on the floor of the pool.

I hold onto an adult's hands, the steps or the side of the pool, then I bend my knees so my shoulders are under the water and I lean my head back until my ears are wet and my eyes are looking up at the sky. I stretch my arms out wide in the shape of a Y and push my feet off the bottom of the pool keeping my legs stretched and straight, remembering to always point my toes and keep my feet just under the surface of the water. I relax and let the water gently hold me. I practice until I can float to the count of 10.

Look at my toes

Bend my knees

Plant my feet

I CAN PANCAKE FLIP & FLOAT!

FLIP

1.2.3

1.2.3

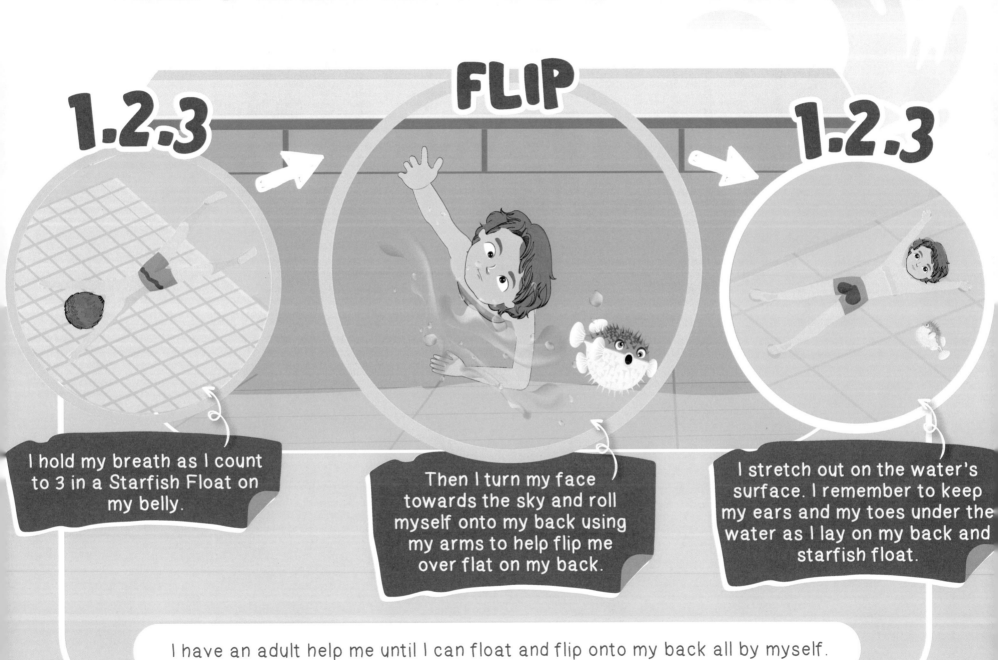

I hold my breath as I count to 3 in a Starfish Float on my belly.

Then I turn my face towards the sky and roll myself onto my back using my arms to help flip me over flat on my back.

I stretch out on the water's surface. I remember to keep my ears and my toes under the water as I lay on my back and starfish float.

I have an adult help me until I can float and flip onto my back all by myself.

12

I CAN TORPEDO STRETCH!

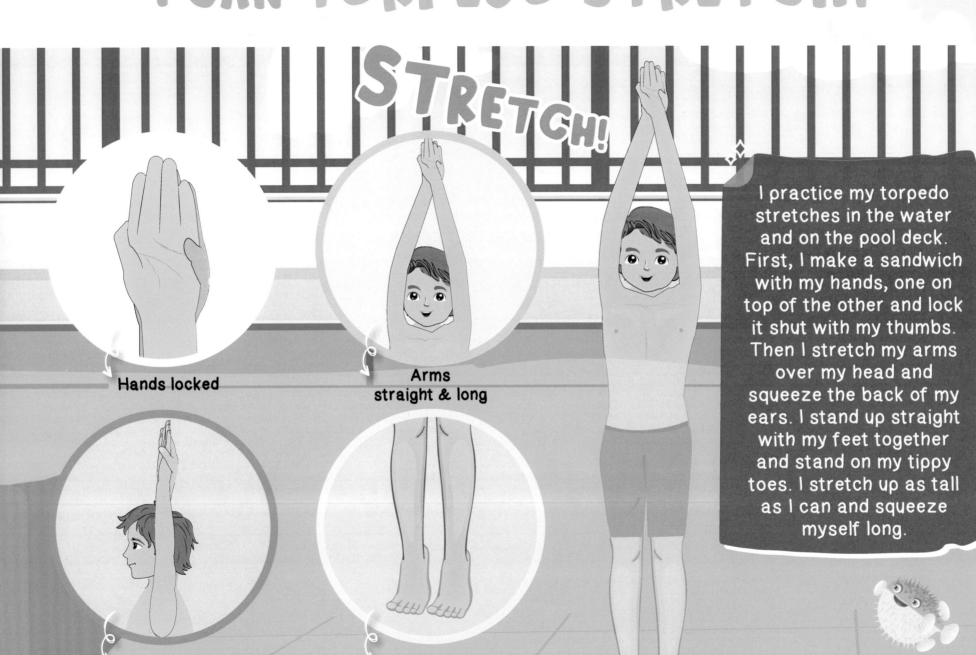

Hands locked

Arms straight & long

STRETCH!

Squeeze ears

Tippy toes

I practice my torpedo stretches in the water and on the pool deck. First, I make a sandwich with my hands, one on top of the other and lock it shut with my thumbs. Then I stretch my arms over my head and squeeze the back of my ears. I stand up straight with my feet together and stand on my tippy toes. I stretch up as tall as I can and squeeze myself long.

I CAN BUNNY CROUCH!

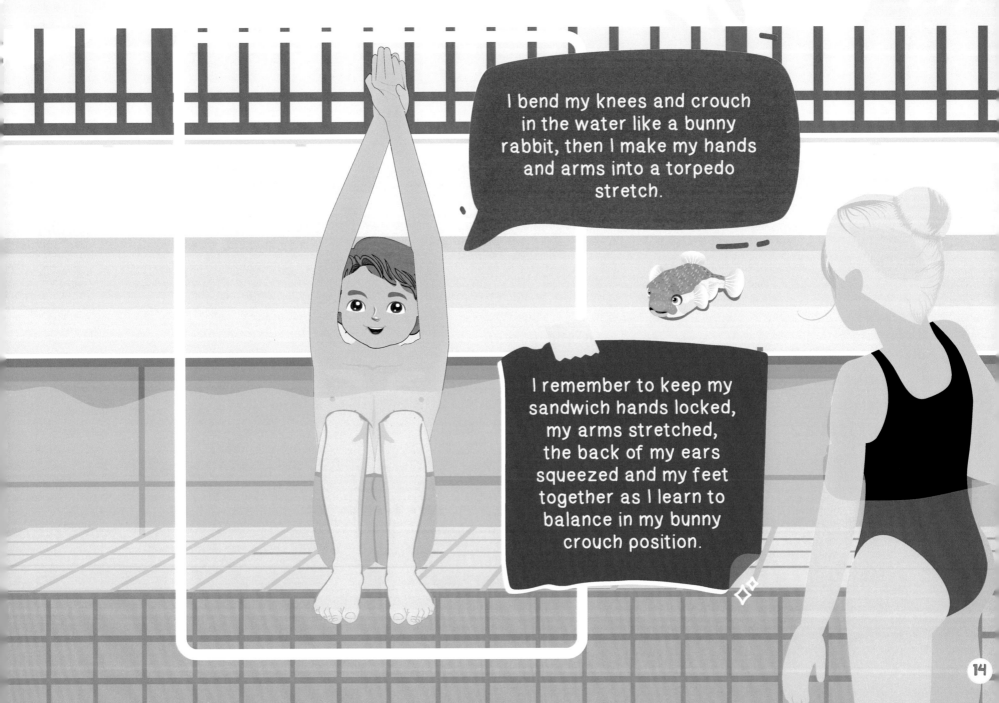

I bend my knees and crouch in the water like a bunny rabbit, then I make my hands and arms into a torpedo stretch.

I remember to keep my sandwich hands locked, my arms stretched, the back of my ears squeezed and my feet together as I learn to balance in my bunny crouch position.

I CAN BUNNY HOP!

3 When my body slows down, I bend my legs and plant my feet on the bottom of the pool. Then, I bunny crouch and push off again across the shallow part of the pool.

1 I bunny crouch on the pool step holding my pufferfish breath as I tilt myself forward.

2 When my face and hands touch the water, I stretch forward and push off with my feet so my legs float to the surface behind me.

I CAN SCISSOR KICK!

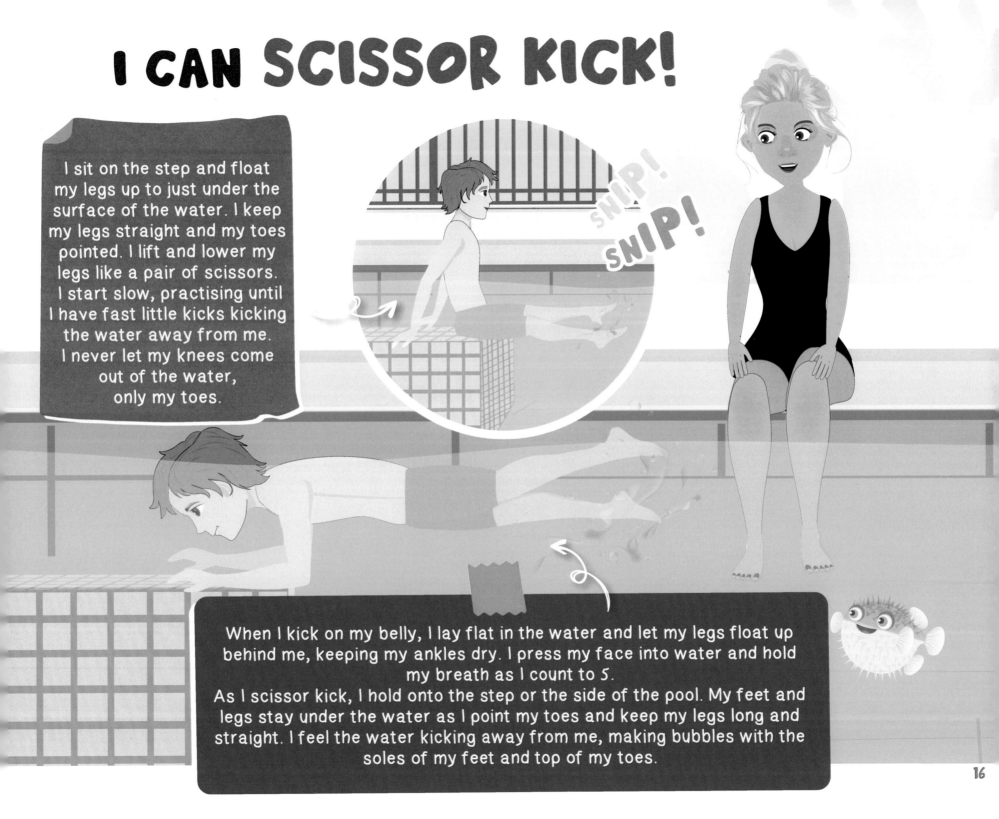

I sit on the step and float my legs up to just under the surface of the water. I keep my legs straight and my toes pointed. I lift and lower my legs like a pair of scissors. I start slow, practising until I have fast little kicks kicking the water away from me. I never let my knees come out of the water, only my toes.

SNIP! SNIP!

When I kick on my belly, I lay flat in the water and let my legs float up behind me, keeping my ankles dry. I press my face into water and hold my breath as I count to 5.
As I scissor kick, I hold onto the step or the side of the pool. My feet and legs stay under the water as I point my toes and keep my legs long and straight. I feel the water kicking away from me, making bubbles with the soles of my feet and top of my toes.

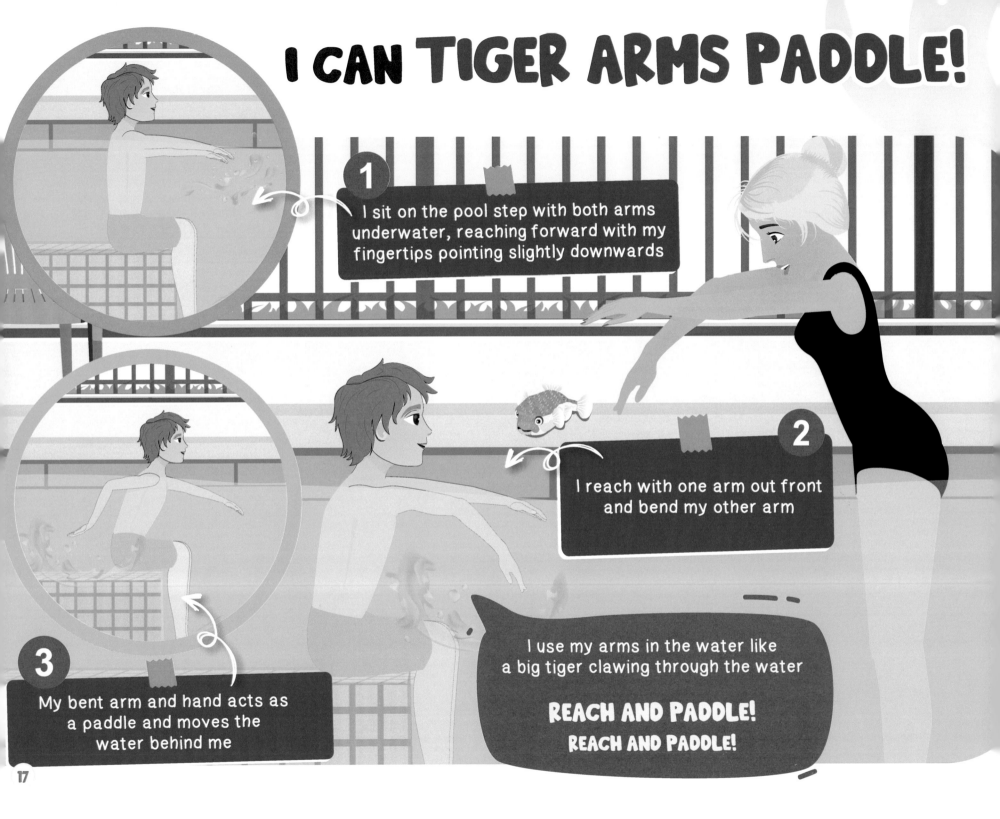

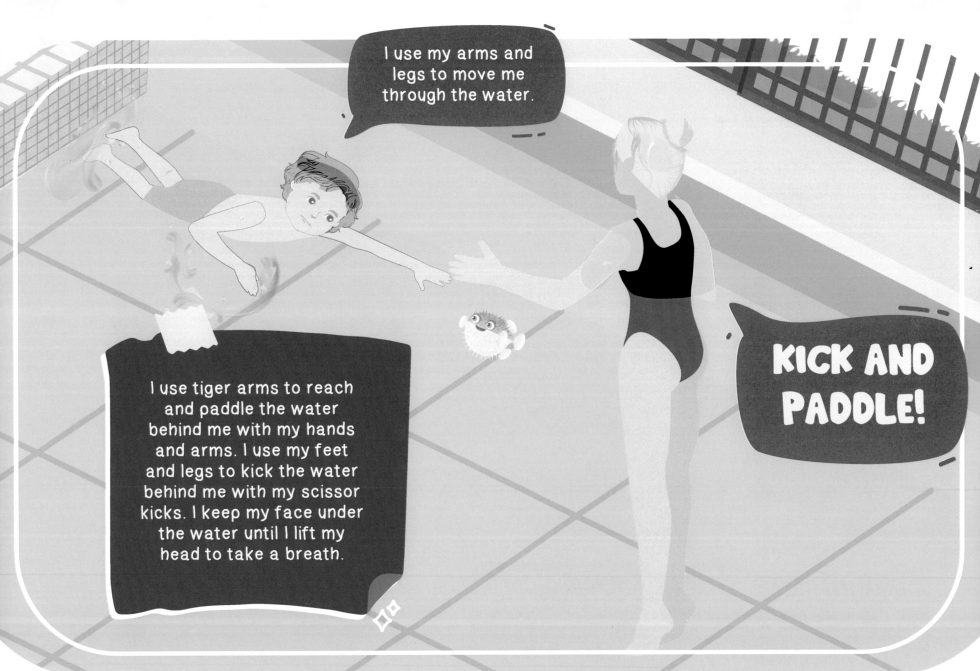

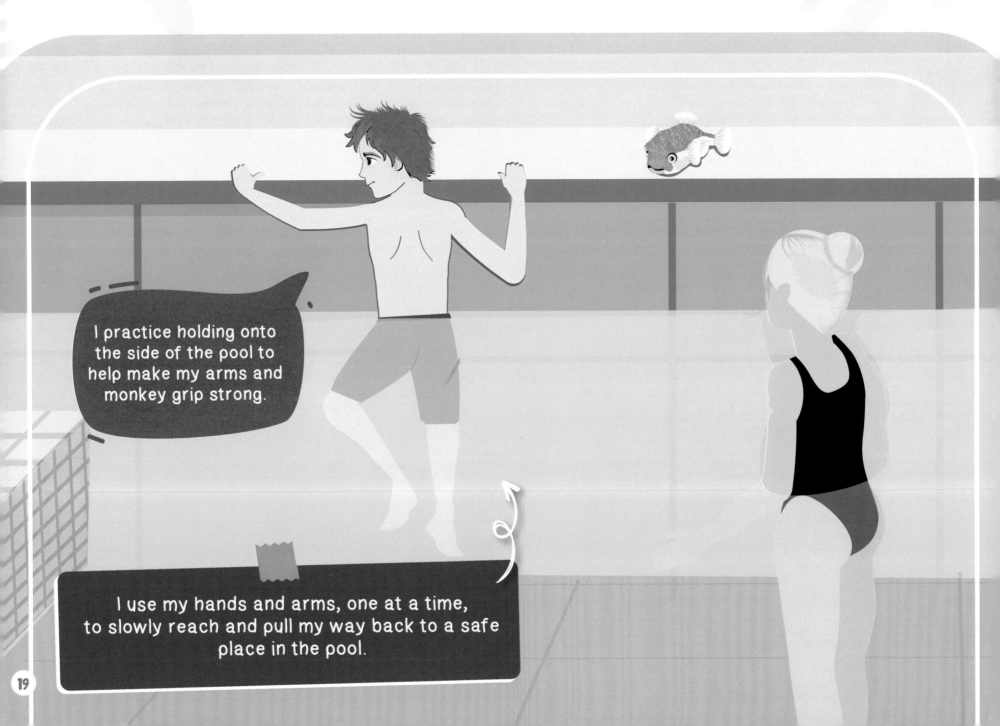

I CAN SAFELY EXIT THE POOL!

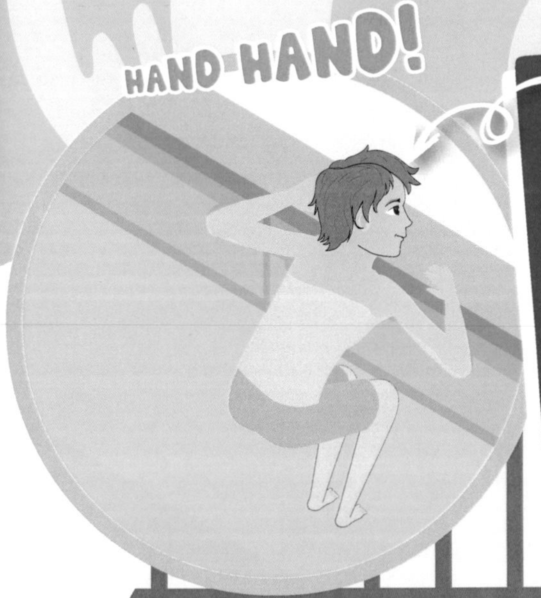

HAND HAND!

To climb out of the pool, I place my hands flat on the pool deck and push down hard to lift my chest out of the water. At the same time. my feet help by using my toes to walk up the pool wall.

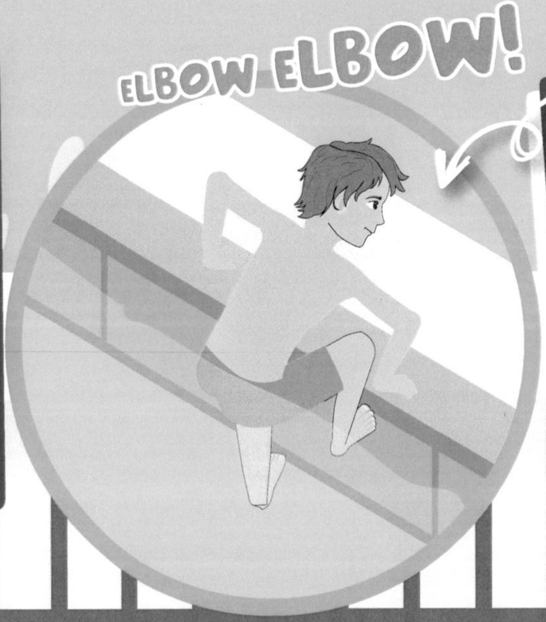

ELBOW ELBOW!

Then, I place one elbow and the other onto the deck and push down hard as I lean forward to lift my leg out using one knee on the pool deck, then my other knee until I am safely out of the pool.

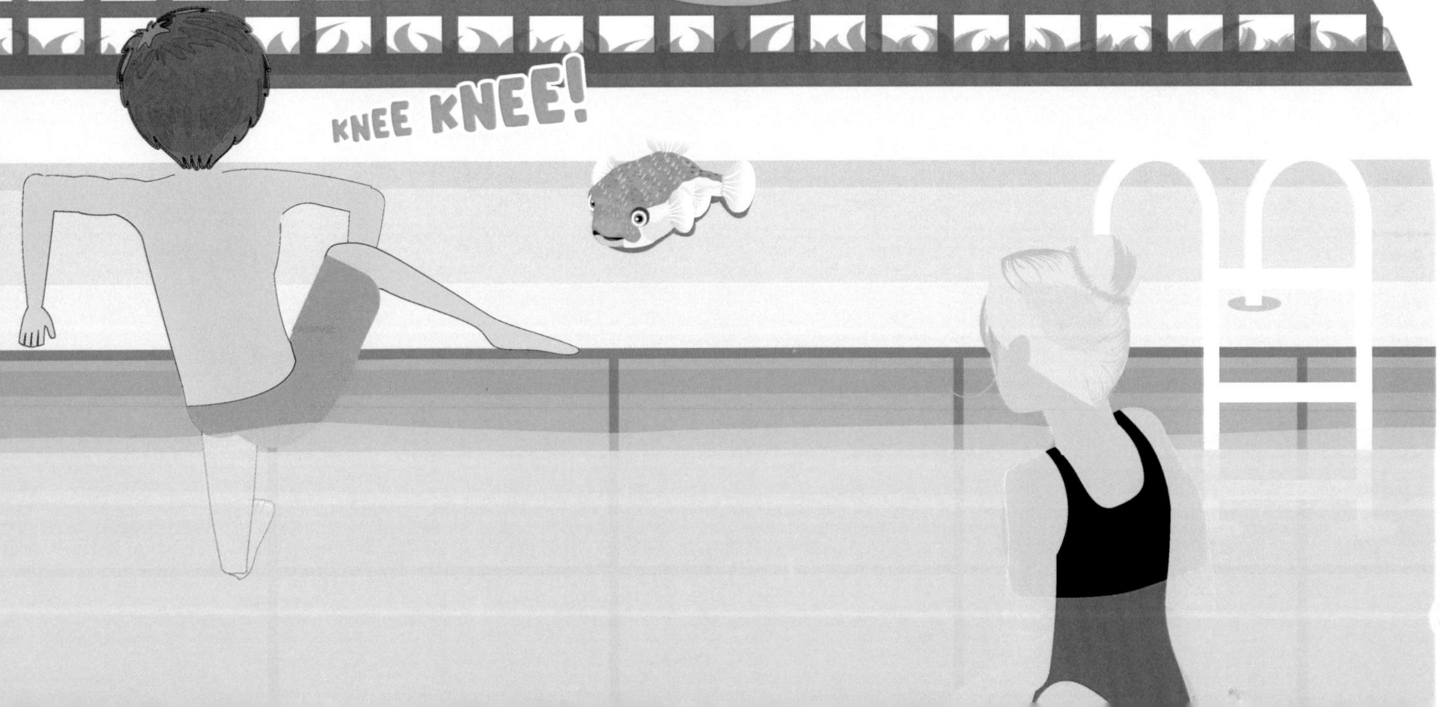

KNEE KNEE!

I practice climbing out of the pool for when there are no steps or ladders nearby.

20

I CAN **SAFELY JUMP** IN THE **POOL!**

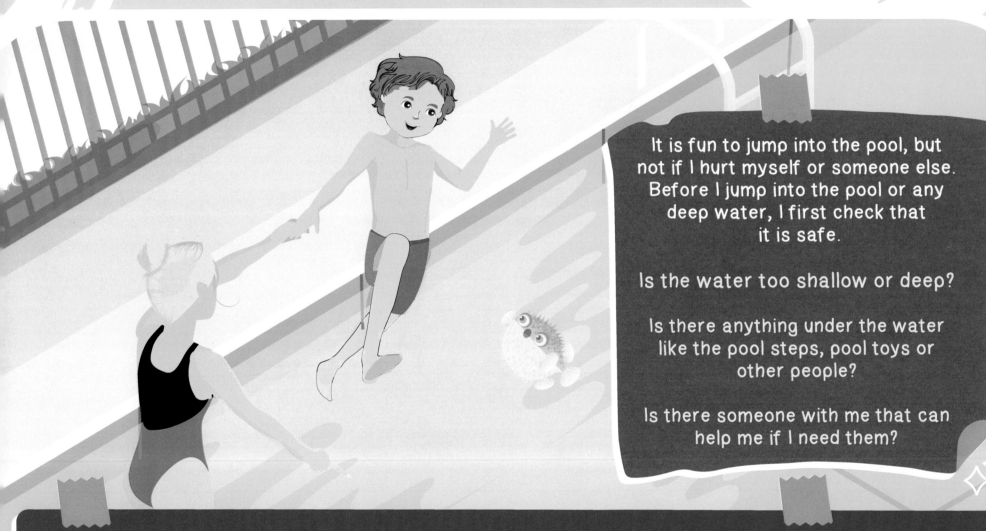

It is fun to jump into the pool, but not if I hurt myself or someone else. Before I jump into the pool or any deep water, I first check that it is safe.

Is the water too shallow or deep?

Is there anything under the water like the pool steps, pool toys or other people?

Is there someone with me that can help me if I need them?

When I first learn to jump safely into the pool, an adult holds my hand and guides me into the pool. When I am ready to do it by myself, I always let an adult know before I jump in.
I put my toes over the edge of the pool deck, bend my knees and push off with my feet. I hold my pufferfish breath as I jump out, feet first, away from the side of the pool so I do not hit my head as I go in. Once I hit the water, I kick and paddle back to the side of the pool and climb out.

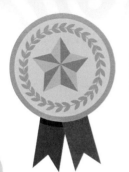

MY ACHIEVEMENTS CHECKLIST

1 I get a little bit better each time I practise my swimming skills.

2 I record my progress using the checklist and a pencil.

3 It reminds me which skills I am really good at and which skills I will need to practise.

4 I know the more I practice the better I will get.

5 When I have practiced and perfected every skill, I know I am ready to move on to Level 2 of Learn to Swim The Australian Way.

	Needs Work	Almost	Perfect
I can safely enter the water			
I can hold my breath			
I can submerge my whole face			
I can bob up and down			
I can crocodile walk			
I can crocodile hold the kickboard			
I can starfish float on my belly			
I can jellyfish float			
I can marshmallow float			
I can teddy bear hug the kickboard			
I can starfish float on my back			
I can pancake flip and float			
I can torpedo stretch			
I can bunny crouch			
I can bunny hop			
I can scissor kick			
I can tiger arms paddle			
I can kick and doggie paddle			
I can monkey-monkey			
I can safely exit the pool			
I can safely jump in the pool			

Lightning Source UK Ltd.
Milton Keynes UK
UKRC031341150922
408912UK00001B/6